Miraculous
Apple Cider Vinegar

How to Use Apple Cider Vinegar for Health Benefits, Beauty, Rapid Weight Loss and Much More

Sarah McMillan

http://sarahmcmillanbooks.com

Table of Contents

Introduction

If you spend a little time on homeopathic message boards or read a lot of health-focused magazines, chances are pretty good you'll hear about apple cider vinegar. In fact, you may already know that a lot of people use apple cider vinegar as a part of their cleaning routine. It's great for cleaning and deodorizing the home, getting rid of cat urine smells on the clothes and eliminating nasty odors in the room. But what you may not know is that apple cider vinegar is not just effective as a cleaning agent, but also so much more.

Apple cider vinegar, commonly referred to as "cider vinegar" or simply as "vinegar," has been an effective treatment for a variety of ailments for centuries. It has been used as everything from a method of lowering blood pressure to cleaning wounds. Applying apple cider vinegar directly to a rash or bug bite has been known to clear them up almost instantly, and stories abound of how apple cider vinegar has helped cure, decrease or keep under control some disease or sickness from people who have used it. You may recall a relative keeping a bottle of apple cider vinegar handy in the kitchen or carrying it along when travelling. It's been around for a very long time and it continues to act as a powerful cleaning agent and source of good health.

Unfortunately, the medical community is not prepared to support the use of apple cider vinegar for medical purposes. On one hand, they stand to lose a lot of patients, as well a lot of money, if everyone started using apple cider vinegar for better health. On the other hand, however, apple cider vinegar is not for everyone. Indeed, some people may be allergic to apple cider vinegar (also referred to as ACV), and it certainly should not be used by someone already on medication. Studies have shown that apple cider vinegar can have harmful effects when taken by someone diagnosed with esophagitis, diabetes, high blood pressure, hypertension and ulcers. Additionally, pregnant women are advised to avoid it. You can read more about cautions to take before using apple cider vinegar at the end of this book.

Even so, while the medical community may use scare tactics or spread a lot of misconceptions about using apple cider vinegar for good health, many studies have shown otherwise. Unfortunately, there is a lot of misunderstanding about how apple cider vinegar works and how it is broken down once digested. This book will clear up those misconceptions and help you better understand how apple cider vinegar works. Also, keep in mind that while it may work for one person, it may not work for you. As with every substance used for medical reasons, results may vary. Start out slowly and see if it brings you the type of benefit you hope to achieve.

If you have been cleared to add apple cider vinegar to your diet, start using it today. Read this book to learn how it can help you achieve good health as well as work as a beauty aid. Apple cider vinegar has benefits both inside and out. It cleanses your body, gets rid of harmful toxins and clears up your skin. You'll also learn how to use it as a detox and how apple cider vinegar can help fight cancer.

Because apple cider vinegar has helped people to experience a lot of health benefits, there have been many misconceptions and warnings being spread around about apple cider vinegar. The medical and scientific community in various parts of the world have taken notice of these pros and cons, and have performed a variety of tests on both animals and humans to see if the ACV does indeed work. Unfortunately, many people have often heard about the tests performed on animals and not on humans, so they may be unaware that tests have also been done on humans. Please note that the exhaustive research done for this book did not rely on results from animal studies. The author has made every effort to hunt down and report on results from tests that have been performed on humans. Unfortunately, there is not a whole lot of press on the human studies, so they may not be so widely known. Don't believe it if someone says "oh, it was only tested on rats" because the author did find studies and tests that included real people. These were the types of evidence used to support what this book shares with you.

If you would like to start using apple cider vinegar as part of your diet or health regimen, you can start doing so at any time. You can use apple cider vinegar in a variety of ways. You can drink it in a diluted drink, top your salads with it or take it as a supplement. You can take it as little or as often as you wish, but be sure to follow the directions included in this book. Consuming too much apple cider vinegar for an extended period of time can cause damage to the stomach lining. You would do well to keep your consumption of it to a minimum. The suggested recipes and directions included in this book come straight from other people who have successfully used it themselves. Ideally, use the suggested recipe or drink mixture that you wish to use the apple cider vinegar for. As an example, you may want to only use apple cider vinegar as an aid to lose weight. The suggestion on how to do so is included in this book. Follow only this suggestion, rather than drinking that particular kind of ACV drink then also taking the supplements or swallowing 2 tablespoons of it a day. Bottom line: Follow the specific instructions included for the type of remedy you seek rather than adding in another recipe or drink mix for other health conditions.

The prospect of buying apple cider vinegar may be intimidating, as there are so many different kinds of vinegar, not just apple cider vinegar, sold on the market, and you may not be sure if you should buy the liquid or the supplement. Follow the suggestions in this book for the type of remedy you seek. When you buy the apple cider vinegar, make sure you buy the right kind to get the best results. It is preferred that you use raw, organic, unfiltered and unpasteurized ACV that contains the "Mother" in it. You can buy this product as a bottle at a grocery store or get the one sold in a jug. You can buy it online, too, if you wish. Store your apple cider vinegar either in the fridge, if you plan to consume it, or in a cool, dark cabinet. Be sure to take note of the expiration date found on the bottle, though it does have a shelf life of 3-5 years. For best results, keep it out of direct sunlight. If you choose to buy the supplements, take note of the expiration date found on the bottle and store it in a cool, ark cabinet.

As with any new product you may be trying to add to your lifestyle or diet, it may take some time for you to get used to using apple cider vinegar. This is especially true if you have not been using it before. You can start off small by making it a morning drink, or you can start adding it to your salads and using it in other recipes. Once you get used to keeping apple cider vinegar as part of a daily routine, you may find it is easier to remember to use it more often and for other purposes. If it helps, print out areas of this book which contain solutions on how to alleviate certain conditions or problems and keep it in plain view in your kitchen or bathroom.

Another way to add and keep apple cider vinegar to your lifestyle is to keep this book handy. Use it often as a reminder of how apple cider vinegar should not be used and to guide you on your path of discovering the miraculous health and beauty benefits of using apple cider vinegar. This book can help you to understand what apple cider vinegar is, how it works, and the many benefits it can mean for you. If you feel it is a good choice to add to your life, keep tabs on your progress and be sure to share the positive results with your friends, family, as well as online. The more good news that is spread about apple cider vinegar, the more we can hopefully dispel the negative talk and misconceptions being spread about it.

Apple cider vinegar may not be the "cure-all" that many tout it to be, but it has definitely shown that it can create a variety of health benefits for many people. It can't hurt to add it to your diet and you may find that it helps make a lot of your recipes and favorite foods just as tasty. Start using it today and see how it can help you on your journey to better health. This book can guide you on your path to getting there and enjoying the many health and beauty benefits of using apple cider vinegar.

What is Apple Cider Vinegar?

Apple cider vinegar has been in use for a very long time. It has been a household staple for centuries and has been used for everything ranging from cleaning kitchen countertops to treating warts. But what exactly is apple cider vinegar? And how is it made?

As the name implies, apple cider vinegar is the vinegar collected from cider or an apple. It is also commonly referred to as "cider vinegar" or "ACV." (You will find it commonly referred to as ACV throughout this book.)

Ever since the discovery of its health benefits, apple cider vinegar has been made commercially available for wider use. Most often, anyone who wants to buy apple cider vinegar need only visit their local grocery store to pick up a bottle. But in the old days, they had to get their apple cider vinegar the hard, old-fashioned way. To get the vinegar, one need only crush up the apples and squeeze out the liquid. Bacteria and yeast are then added to start the fermentation process. The natural sugars from the apples will be converted to alcohol as a result. The acidic bacteria converts the alcohol into vinegar. This will give the liquid its sour taste when fermentation is complete.

Essentially, apple cider vinegar comes straight from the apples. It becomes a "cider" because of the juice it is turned into and a "vinegar" because of the sour taste it develops. If the ACV is unpasteurized or if it's an organic brand, it will likely contain "mother of vinegar," which is a substance consisting of cellulose and acetic acid bacteria as a result of the fermentation process. This is the "meaty" part of the apples and is referred to as "the Mother" in homeopathic communities discussing ACV, as well as when it is labeled on the bottle sold in stores. It is called the "Mother" because it can be used to create more apple cider vinegar.

Even after the apples are crushed, some of the natural source of pectin from the apple may be present in apple cider vinegar. The pectin has been useful in treating a variety of ailments because it acts as a natural source of fiber. There are other types of vitamins and minerals which exist in ACV, as well.

Vitamins present in apple cider vinegar:

- Vitamin B1,

- Vitamin B2

- Vitamin B6

- Biotin (Vitamin H)

- Folic acid (Vitamin B9 or Vitamin Bc)

- Niacin (Vitamin B3)

- Pantothenic acid (Vitamin B5)

- Vitamin C

In addition to the many vitamins found in apple cider vinegar, there are also many different minerals present. They are not in copious amounts or amounts large enough to have much health or digestive benefit, but the minerals in apple cider vinegar are still useful in their own ways.

Minerals present in apple cider vinegar:

- Sodium

- Phosphorous

- Potassium

- Calcium

- Iron

- Magnesium

Given its nutritional content and overall dose of power-packed vitamins, it's no wonder people have been using apple cider vinegar for health reasons. As you'll learn in the next chapter, however, there are a great deal of other uses for apple cider vinegar. Some of these alternative uses just may surprise you.

The Many Uses for Apple Cider Vinegar

For the longest time, people have been using apple cider vinegar for a variety of reasons. It's been a staple in many recipes (including as a salad dressing) and useful for cleaning purposes. But did you know there are other things you can use apple cider vinegar for?

Below is a list of alternative uses for apple cider vinegar. While these uses have worked for some people, they may not work for everyone. You may need to give the method included some time to work or wait a little longer for the desired effect. As with all methods, try it out a little bit at a time first, or try it on a small, unnoticeable area.

Odor neutralizer

Apple cider vinegar has quite a kick for taste, but it also kicks as an odor-buster as well. If you have a pungent odor in any room of the home, you can leave out a bowl of apple cider vinegar where the odor is strongest. No need to warm it or add anything else. Just pour it into a shallow bowl and leave it out until the odor is gone.

Weed killer

Want a natural way to kill the weeds lurking in your garden? Go after them with apple cider vinegar! Just pour the ACV onto the weeds until their lack of growth is noticeable. Remove the dead weeds. Make the soil weed-resistent by combining 10 ounces of apple cider vinegar with 10 gallons of water and spray over the area. Bye-bye, weeds!

Natural flea killer

If your dog or cat has a flea problem, you can nip it in the bud with apple cider vinegar! This has been known to help pet owners rid their animals of fleas, but do discuss it with your vet before going any further. If the vet gives the okay, combine one part of apple cider vinegar to one part of water and mix it well. Rub it into your animal friend's fur, making sure it gets contact with the skin. You should see results instantly.

Natural B.O. buster

Another type of odor the apple cider vinegar will attack? Body odor. You can use apple cider vinegar as a natural deodorant and the best part is that it will dissolve into your skin so you won't be going around with the smell of the vinegar so obvious. Just rub some of it under the arms or where needed and take on the day without the B.O.

Relief from itchy skin

If you've got an itch that just won't seem to go away, try applying apple cider vinegar to the area. Some medicines may not work as effectively as they claim and dealing with itchy skin can be a nightmare. Just use apple cider vinegar for relief and take comfort that you're using a more natural product to take care of that itch.

A natural energy drink

While it's not a good idea to drink raw apple cider vinegar, as it can irritate the throat, you can mix it with other things and drink it down just fine. In fact, combining apple cider vinegar with other things will create an instant energy drink that will have you experiencing a fresh burst of energy. Combine two teaspoons of apple cider vinegar with two cups of water and add a bit of honey for taste. Drink it down and be ready to take on the world all over again!

Digestive aid for beans

For anyone who enjoys eating beans but does not appreciate the digestive side effects, apple cider vinegar can be of help. When you soak the beans, be sure to add one or two tablespoons of apple cider vinegar to the water. Let the beans soak for 18-24 hours before cooking.

Cleaning uses

It's no secret that apple cider vinegar works just as good as commercial cleaning products. The trick is to use it properly.

One thing you can do is create a "multi-purpose cleaning spray" with apple cider vinegar. Mix together one part of apple cider vinegar with one part water in a spray bottle then use to clean countertops, tiled floors, cabinets, etc. You can also add two cups of apple cider vinegar to the toilet, let sit overnight then flush for a bright clean. For glass surfaces, combine ½ cup of apple cider vinegar with 1 cup of water then spray to clean microwaves, windows and mirrors. Need to get rid of lime build-up in your tea kettle? Pour 1 cup of apple cider vinegar into your tea kettle and let it sit overnight. Next, boil it for 10 minutes, then rinse with fresh water. Use apple cider vinegar to clean your shower drain, as well. Combine 1 cup of apple cider vinegar with ½ cup of salt, ¼ cup of baking soda and 4 cups of boiling water. Pour this down your shower drain, wait 15 minutes then "rinse" it by pouring 4 cups of boiling water down the drain again.

Natural produce wash

We all know the importance of giving vegetables a good scrub before eating or cooking them, and stores happily push vegetable washes our way. But you can DIY with apple cider vinegar! Simply add 4 tablespoons of ACV to 1 gallon of water and scrub away the dirt and grime on your fruits and veggies.

Natural ant repellant

An ant infestation can be a nightmare, but apple cider vinegar can help you combat these pests. Simply spray raw apple cider vinegar over their tracks to eliminate the scent ants leave there to find their way into your house. Spray it on cracks and anywhere else ants can get in to keep those bugs out.

As you add apple cider vinegar to your lifestyle, you may discover it can have other uses, as well. There's no limit on the natural cleaning and health benefits of apple cider vinegar. Some of its other benefits remain undiscovered. This chapter has introduced you to the known uses of apple cider vinegar that has worked for a lot of people. Use apple cider vinegar for any one of these needs and experience for yourself just why they call it a "miracle product."

Health Benefits of Apple Cider Vinegar

Apple cider vinegar has been a valuable cleaning solution, but did you know that it can help alleviate or cure a whole host of health problems? Many people have used ACV to find relief from a variety of ailments and chances are good it can help you, too. The next time you suffer from one health condition or another, think about using apple cider vinegar to find relief.

Here are the many ways in which apple cider vinegar can provide you with health benefits. Please note that while this has worked for many people, it may not work for you. Still, it's worth a try. If you are unsure about using apple cider vinegar for health remedies, consult with your doctor before trying any one of these methods.

Weight loss

Apple cider vinegar has helped a number of people lose weight. It takes 12 weeks of using ACV for a weight loss program to notice any results. People who used it in such studies lost more weight in 3 months than those who did not use it. There is some proof that consuming apple cider vinegar activates a gene that assists in weight loss. Additionally, apple cider vinegar has helped to boost metabolism and it destroys fat. If you wish to use apple cider vinegar for weight loss, keep in mind that you will also need to exercise and watch what you eat while using ACV. We will discuss how to use apple cider vinegar as part of a weight loss program in a later chapter.

Lowering blood sugar

Apple cider vinegar has definitely been shown to help people lower their blood sugar. This has been helpful in preventing diabetes as well as managing health conditions associated with high blood sugar levels. Remember to talk with your doctor before using ACV for this purpose. If your doctor gives you the okay to use ACV for controlling your blood sugar levels, simply add two tablespoons of ACV to a 16-ounce glass of water and drink with your meals twice a day.

Lowering blood pressure

There has been proof that apple cider vinegar can assist in lowering blood pressure. Some folks have found that this actually works. The thing to do is add 1 tablespoon of raw apple cider vinegar to a glass of water, as well as 1 tablespoon of raw honey (not commercial honey) and stir it all together. Drink this three times a day and you'll start noticing a change in your blood pressure in a few weeks.

Boosting metabolism

Another health benefit from apple cider vinegar? It'll help kick your metabolism into gear, which will also add to the weight loss benefit mentioned earlier. Simply add a couple of teaspoons of ACV to a glass of water and drink before each meal.

Treating high cholesterol

Apple cider vinegar has also been proven to fight high cholesterol in both animals and humans. High cholesterol can lead to hypertension and heart disease. Just as little as 0.5 ounces a day is enough to keep low density cholesterol (LDL) at low levels. Here again is where drinking it in your water three times a day can help.

Relief from acid reflux

If you've chosen to have a drink of water with two tablespoons of apple cider vinegar stirred in, you're on the right path to beating heartburn, gas and bloating. You can also get this benefit by adding a tablespoon of ACV to a cup of tea. Drink before meals or as soon as you start experiencing the symptoms of heartburn.

Allergy relief

Apple cider vinegar has helped many people suffering from allergies find relief. The common allergy symptoms such as shortness of breath, nasal congestion, coughing, sneezing, watery eyes and itchy skin have all been cleared up when someone suffering from such allergy symptoms began adding apple cider vinegar to their diet. You can add 2 tablespoons of

ACV to water and drink it with your meals, or add the same amount to tea or apple juice. It's fine to add honey for flavoring, as well. Additionally, inhaling the steam from apple cider vinegar can help alleviate allergy attacks. You will learn how to achieve this affect later in this chapter.

Help for sinus problems

The vitamins and minerals found in apple cider vinegar are helpful in clearing up sinus problems. Apple cider vinegar also contains a high pH level, another tool in fighting sinus problems. People suffering from such problems don't get the relief they need when using over-the-counter products; instead, apple cider vinegar has actually been the better choice to help such people. You can take ACV capsules or mix the liquid with water then drink twice a day to get this benefit. Or, inhale the steam. To do so, combine ½ cup of apple cider vinegar with ½ cup of water in a pan and warm it up on the stove for a few minutes. Turn off the heat then inhale the steam wafting up from the pan. You will need to do this for a few minutes and as often as possible to get relief from sinus problems.

Help cure yeast infections

Because of its high acidic level and level of pH, apple cider vinegar is useful in combatting yeast infections. It is one of nature's strongest antibiotics and can kill excess yeast in your body. It has also been known to strengthen the immune system and fight candida, which is the bad bacteria that can cause an infection. To get this benefit, make apple cider vinegar a regular part of your diet. You can drink it with water or sprinkle it on your salads. You can also take ACV as a capsule or tablet. Additionally, you can use it as a douche treatment by combining 3 tablespoons of ACV with 4 quarts of warm water and using it twice a day. Finally, you can soak in an ACV bath by adding 3 cups of ACV to the bath water and soaking for at least 15 minutes twice a day. While you are treating this condition, avoid sweets until the infection is gone and add more yogurt to your diet, as well.

Help for respiratory problems

Apple cider vinegar is a strong bacteria-killer. In fact, one kind of bacteria it has been known to kill are the kind found in your chest and throat that causes mucus. When experiencing chest or throat problems, mix one tablespoon of apple cider vinegar into a glass of water and drink it down. It should help instantly.

Help for de-stressing

Combat stress with apple cider vinegar? It can be done! Research has shown that people with high levels of stress seemed to feel better after consuming apple cider vinegar. Either eat a salad with the vinegar as a dressing or drink it in your water. The enzymes in ACV will alleviate the symptoms associated with stress.

Alleviating constipation and IBS

Not only is apple cider vinegar a natural antibiotic in many cases, but it is also a natural laxative. The natural pectin from the apples is a water soluble fiber, which can help cure constipation. It has also been known to alleviate Irritable Bowel Syndrome (IBS), a more painful form of constipation. For constipation relief, mix 2 tablespoons of ACV with 1 tablespoon of raw or manuka honey and mix together in a glass of warm water. Drink on an empty stomach in the morning as well as a half hour before bedtime. Continue to drink until the constipation is gone. For relief from IBS, add 2 tablespoons of ACV to a glass of water and drink it with your lunch and dinner. For best results, do not drink it on an empty stomach.

Help for mouth disorders

Apple cider vinegar can help anyone with mouth problems, ranging from a sore throat to bad breath. To treat a sore throat, add 1 tablespoon of ACV to a glass of warm water and gargle every hour until you feel relief. Adults may also need to swallow a tablespoonful of ACV after gargling. To combat bad breath, use ACV as a mouthwash. Simply combine a teaspoon of it with ¼ cup of water and use as a mouth rinse after brushing your teeth. This will kill odor-causing bacteria as well as prevent the build-up of plaque.

Getting rid of warts

If you want a natural remedy to get rid of a wart, look no further than apple cider vinegar. All you need to do is soak a cotton pad in ACV then apply it over the wart. Apply a bandage to keep it in place. Leave this on overnight then remove in the morning. After a week, the wart will dry up and disappear.

Help for gallbladder problems

Many people suffering from gallbladder attacks as a result of gallstones have found relief from the pain thanks to apple cider vinegar. To use for such situations, add 2 tablespoons of ACV to 1 cup of organic apple juice and drink it down. You should feel relief in 20-30 minutes.

Diabetes

Studies on people with Type 2 Diabetes have shown that apple cider vinegar can be helpful in fighting the disease. Participants in the study were given solution containing five teaspoons of vinegar, five teaspoons of water, and one teaspoon of saccharin two minutes before consuming a high-carb meal. They were tested 30 minutes before and 60 minutes after the meal, and doctors were surprised to see a drop in insulin levels in the people who ingested the vinegar solution.

Treating anemia

Anemia occurs when there is not enough iron in the body. This can cause lack of strength, fatigue and dizziness. Aside from adding more iron to your diet, you can also combat anemia by using apple cider vinegar. To use, swallow a tablespoon of ACV in the morning on an empty stomach. It will take up to a month to restore sufficient iron to your body and get rid of anemia.

Treating gout

Apple cider vinegar has helped many people suffering from gout. Apple cider vinegar has powerful enzymes and it is a strong anti-inflammatory liquid. It helps blood circulation in the joints and alleviates swelling. It may take a while before there are noticeable results, but given the added health benefits of drinking ACV, it's a good idea to add it to your diet and get started on fighting this other major health problem. Simply add two tablespoons of ACV and one teaspoon of raw honey to a glass of water and drink it twice a day.

Arthritis

Another way apple cider vinegar has helped with a health condition is combatting arthritis. Mix 1 tablespoon of apple cider vinegar into water and add a tablespoon of honey. Drink first thing in the morning.

Athlete's foot

Athlete's foot occurs because of fungus on the feet. To get relief, add one part of apple cider vinegar to three parts of water and soak your feet in the water for at least 30 minutes.

The list of the many health benefits associated with apple cider vinegar could go on and on. What better argument do you need for adding it to your diet? Even if you don't have any of the health issues listed here, adding a couple of tablespoons of apple cider vinegar to a glass of water and drinking it a couple of times a day is a great health habit because it will make your immune system stronger and enable your body to fight off infection. Think about adding apple cider vinegar to your diet and watch how healthier and stronger you'll start feeling.

Apple Cider Vinegar for Men's Health

Apple cider vinegar has a variety of health benefits for both men and women. It has been shown to fight dandruff, improve skin health and cure hiccups. However, studies have shown that ACV has health benefits exclusively for men. Men have found relief from certain ailments after they began using ACV, and the added benefit is that including apple cider vinegar in their diets has helped them achieve the other health benefits such as a stronger immune system and a boost in energy.

Before using any one of these treatments for these conditions, talk with your doctor first. Keep in mind that apple cider vinegar is highly acidic and should never be applied to the skin or digestive tract without first being combined with another liquid, such as water. You can try using one of these treatments in addition to a treatment recommended by your doctor, but remember to follow instructions and don't add too much ACV to your mixture. It may take some time before you notice results so give the treatment time to work. If you are unsure about using any one of these suggested treatments, discuss it with your doctor or do a bit of research about it first. Results may vary.

Male Yeast Infection

Yes, men get yeast infections, too. And apple cider vinegar has proven to help get rid of it! To use, draw a warm low bath, with enough water to cover the legs and genitals. Add 2 cups of apple cider vinegar to the water. Soak for at least 30 minutes. If there is foreskin, it should be pulled back.

Male Menopause (Andropause)

Men also experience menopause, but unlike women, this condition, which can strike after age 50, does not affect all men. Symptoms men may experience during this time are penile shrinkage, lack of erection, low sex drive, genital warts, hot flashes, mood swings, irritability and depression. Apple cider vinegar has been used in creating an herbal "tincture" that goes by the name "Horny Goat Weed" and it is available in herbal stores as well as online. It has been found to help men going through this to experience an increased sex drive.

Treatment for gonorrhea

Soak a bandage in apple cider vinegar mixed with coconut oil. Apply to the affected areas of the genitals, wrapping bandage securely. Leave on until condition clears; change bandage when needed. Also, mix one tablespoon of apple cider vinegar into five cups of warm water and bathe the affected area daily.

Erectile dysfunction

Some men have experienced success in eliminating erectile dysfunction after they began taking the ACV supplement, which is sold in herbal stores. Apple cider vinegar repairs damaged blood vessels and nerve fibers in the penis, and it also has been proven to reduce the swelling of the prostate gland. A bonus is that it may even boost testosterone levels. Results are obvious usually after a few days of taking the supplement.

Peptic ulcer

Anyone can get an ulcer, but peptic ulcers are more common in men. Peptic ulcers result when the bacteria *Helicobacter pylori* creates a hole in the stomach lining. Men often shrug off this discomfort, calling it a "sour stomach" or indigestion. You can treat it with apple cider vinegar. Simply mix together two parts water and one part apple cider vinegar and drink it as soon as the discomfort sets in. It may take a few weeks for the ulcer to clear up.

Baldness

Women and men can both go bald, but baldness happens more commonly in men. Apple cider vinegar can help restore hair growth! Add 4 ounces of ACV to 4 ounces of water. Add 10 drops of sage essential oil. Pour this onto your hair, ensuring it comes into contact with your scalp. Wrap hair in a towel and allow it to sit for a half hour. Remove the towel then rinse and wash hair. Do this once a week to ensure you maintain good, strong hair growth and avoid balding areas.

Prostate cancer

Apple cider vinegar has proven to be a good cancer fighter, but one of the cancers it can combat is cancer of the prostate. Studies have shown that ACV has slowed the growth of cancer cells in the prostate. For best results, take ACV as a supplement.

Many men may shy away from "home remedies" but using apple cider vinegar for male-related health issues has been proven to work. Consider picking up a bottle of the organic apple cider sold in stores, with the "Mother" contained in it, or use it as a supplement and watch just how much of a positive change it can create for your health.

Using Apple Cider Vinegar for Pain Relief

Apple cider vinegar has anti-inflammatory benefits. It has been known to reduce swelling, improve blood flow and alleviate pain. In fact, it was used as an antiseptic during the Civil War. Many people try to dispel the pain-killing benefits of apple cider vinegar, but for many, it has worked.

Before using apple cider vinegar for pain relief, be sure to consult with your doctor first. Look into your options and see if this is the best choice for you. Remember that one person's cure may be another person's placebo, so keep in mind that not all of these suggestions may work in your situation. You may also need to give the solution some time to work. It can take days, weeks or months before you notice any pain relief from the suggested use.

For most cases, the best way to use apple cider vinegar for pain relief is as follows: Add 2 tablespoons of apple cider vinegar and 2 teaspoons of organic honey to a glass of water or juice and drink twice a day before meals. In some cases, it will need to be used differently, depending on the type of pain. In those cases, information about the effective use is included. Wait a few days to see results.

Some people with digestive problems may experience intestinal pain or discomfort after eating certain foods. This is where apple cider vinegar can come in handy. Because it contains pectin, apple cider vinegar aids digestion and alleviates intestinal cramping. This will also help prevent the pain associated with diarrhea and alleviate the discomfort of defecation.

Hiccups are an annoying disruption a lot of people experience every once in a while. If the hiccups get to be too intense or last for too long, it can cause chest pain. To get rid of the hiccups, quickly down a shot of raw apple cider vinegar. While it is strongly recommended that you never drink the apple cider vinegar without diluting it first, the rare occurrence of hiccups makes it okay to use raw apple cider vinegar for just such a purpose. Done only once and on very rare occasions, it will not harm your teeth, throat or stomach compared to constant consumption of the vinegar. However, you can chase this down with a glass of water, if you wish.

Itchy skin that lasts for too long can cause pain on your skin, as well. It is also a real hassle to deal with an area of itchy skin that doesn't seem to heal. To stop the itch, simply rub a small amount of apple cider vinegar over the area.

Tired of dealing with joint pain? Apple cider vinegar can help you find relief. Simply stir a half cup of apple cider vinegar into 3 cups of apple juice and add 2 cups of grape juice. Drink 8 ounces of this every morning.

Pain associated with a hangover? Apple cider vinegar can help. Mix 2 tablespoons of apple cider vinegar with 1 tablespoon of honey in a glass of water and drink it down.

Got a sore throat? A sore throat, or any kind of throat pain, will be lessened by apple cider vinegar. Simply gargle with it twice a day until the throat pain goes away.

Pain from a sunburn can be really unpleasant. Apple cider vinegar can alleviate this pain, too. To use apple cider vinegar for treating a painful sunburn, add 2 tablespoons of apple cider vinegar to 2 cups of cold water. Soak a washcloth in the solution and apply it to the sunburned area. Leave it on for a little while. If possible, after you remove the cloth, apply area vera to the area. Alternatively, you can soak in a healing bath by adding 2 cups of apple cider vinegar to cool bath water. Stay in the bath for at least 30 minutes. After you gently dab the area dry, apply aloe vera to the area.

Because of its many healing properties, apple cider vinegar has been helpful in offering pain relief. The best part is that it can be taken orally or applied as a diluted solution to the affected area. The next time you want a natural source of pain relief, consider reaching for the apple cider vinegar and get rid of whatever pain is ailing you.

How Apple Cider Vinegar Fights Cancer

Probably one of the most hotly debated topics about the healing benefits of apple cider vinegar is whether or not it can cure cancer. When most proponents of homeopathic medicine talk about apple cider vinegar and cancer, there is a lot of focus on how it "heals" it. You'll find a lot of "miracle stories" of how apple cider vinegar helped many people beat cancer.

The truth is that apple cider vinegar does not "cure" cancer per se, but it does help fight cancer. It has certainly been an effective tool in fighting the "C" and if you're interested in using apple cider vinegar as part of your cancer treatment, it's definitely a viable choice.

What is it about apple cider vinegar that makes it useful in fighting cancer? There are actually two reasons why it is certainly a smart tool to use.

One of the arguments or why apple cider vinegar can help fight cancer is that it contains Vitamin C. Vitamin C has been proven to inhibit the growth of tumors.

Another argument is that it creates a more alkalinic environment in the body. Cancer cannot live in an alkaline environment, and people who consume apple cider vinegar will eventually boost their body's alkalinity. Apple cider vinegar may be highly acidic, yes, but once ingested and digested, the body will create a highly alkalinic ash that will neutralize the acid. Thus, it will not end up being such an acidic substance in the digestive system. Unfortunately, this beneficial transformation which takes place once apple cider vinegar is digested is not so widely known. Many people see apple cider vinegar as "acidic" and immediately pass it over as a way of benefiting their health. More people should understand that the acidic quality of apple cider vinegar changes after digestion and this change is actually good for the body.

There are many stories out there of apple cider vinegar helping to fight cancer. You can talk with your doctor about this option, but unfortunately, the medical community does not support using apple cider vinegar as a form of treatment in the fight against cancer. Sadly, there is a lot of money doctors stand to make in cancer treatment, so they are not entirely prepared to support a homeopathic remedy that could mean they'll lose a profit. It is up to you whether or not you want to use apple cider vinegar as a method to fight cancer. Do your research and see what works for you.

That said, the types of cancer that apple cider vinegar has proven to help fight are as follows:

- Breast cancer

- Colon cancer

- Esophageal cancer

- Gastrointestinal cancer

- Geosophical Cancer

- Prostate cancer

- Skin cancer

Ultimately, apple cider vinegar can be beneficial in the fight against cancer. It has been proven to shrink tumors and kill cancer cells. As mentioned previously, it also reduces swelling associated with prostate cancer and it also helps fight skin cancer. There may be many opponents out there putting down the cancer-fighting benefits of apple cider vinegar, but when held up against the many stories of people who have beat cancer thanks to the help of ACV, what more do you stand to lose? Cancer is a vicious killer that can kill very quickly and you would do well to use whatever forms of treatment are at your disposal in putting a stop to it.

If you choose to include apple cider vinegar in your treatment of cancer, the best method has been to stir two tablespoons of the cider vinegar into a glass of water and add 2 teaspoons of raw honey. Drink this twice daily and eventually you will notice results. It's also a good idea to include foods such as salads with apple cider vinegar dressing or pickled eggs into your diet.

Think about including apple cider vinegar in your diet as a way to fight cancer and watch how it can help you win the battle.

Apple Cider Vinegar for Heart Health

Many proponents of apple cider vinegar have personally witnessed just how helpful it can be to boost heart health. Apple cider vinegar has been used for medicinal purposes for ages and it has shown time and again that it is one of nature's most potent fighters against heart disease, as well as other problems affecting the heart. It prevents damage to cells from free radicals, which can lead to heart disease. The pectin in ACV helps keep levels of cholesterol low. High cholesterol levels can eventually cause heart disease.

There have been studies of how apple cider vinegar helps heart health in rats, yes, but there have also been studies including people. The results of these studies were promising. Those who used apple cider vinegar compared to those who did not, or those who were given a different kind of vinegar, were the ones who came out with positive results in boosting their heart health.

Apple cider vinegar works in a variety of ways to ensure good heart health in people who consume it. For one thing, it lowers cholesterol, which can ensure prevention of heart disease and stroke. It cleans out the arteries, so that the heart can continue to work effectively. It lowers blood sugar levels, which helps prevent diabetes, which can further lead to heart disease. It would seem the myriad health benefits of apple cider vinegar come together to achieve one goal: Making sure you continue to enjoy good heart health.

It will take approximately 8 to 10 weeks before you'll notice any heart health benefits of consuming apple cider vinegar. Give it some time and, meanwhile, enjoy the other added benefits of consuming apple cider vinegar, such as clearer skin and a boost in energy.

There are two ways you can achieve the heart health benefits of apple cider vinegar. Most studies done with people only included apple cider vinegar used as a food and not as a supplement, so consider adding it to your diet instead of swallowing the capsules. The two methods employed in these studies are as follow:

Put it on your salad

A study of people who ate salads with vinegar dressing six times a week showed that they were at lower risk for heart disease.

Swallow it directly

Swallow a couple of spoonfuls of apple cider vinegar a day. If the taste is too much for you to tolerate, wash it down with water or add organic honey.

In addition to using apple cider vinegar to improve your heart health, it is a good idea to practice other healthy habits, as well. Don't assume that swallowing two spoons of apple cider vinegar a day will be enough for your heart health and think it's okay to continue being a couch potato and eating fried foods. You'll need to implement other habits, too, such as proper diet, exercise and drinking a lot of water. If you're a smoker, try to kick the habit.

Make sure you are not trying to use apple cider vinegar while you are also taking heart medication. Studies have found that when combined, the apple cider vinegar can actually have a negative effect on the medication. It may not even allow the medication to work properly. Talk with your doctor first to find out if you can consume apple cider vinegar while on your medication.

Naysayers may claim that apple cider vinegar is not as good a choice in combatting heart disease or other heart problems, but the results of studies including humans pretty much speak for themselves. Think about including apple cider vinegar in your diet if you want to have good heart health. If anything, you'll be consuming a natural product shown to have a variety of health benefits without causing any damage to your heart health routine.

Apple Cider Vinegar and AIDS

Considering that apple cider vinegar has a whole host of health benefits for a lot of people who suffer from a variety of health problems, one can only question if apple cider vinegar can be helpful in the fight against AIDS.

The Acquired Immune Deficiency Syndrome (AIDS) virus is a worldwide killer that has taken the lives of millions. A person normally contracts AIDS from the Human Immunodeficiency Virus, known as "HIV." A person can get HIV from unprotected sex with an infected partner, through the transmission of breast milk from someone who is HIV-positive, and by physical contact with an HIV-positive person who has an open wound. Once a person is diagnosed as HIV-positive, they may eventually acquire full-blown AIDS. During the time they are HIV-positive, they may experience several negative health conditions. With their immune system severely impaired because of HIV, they are more susceptible to infections, disease and crippling ailments that could affect them on a much worse level than that of a healthy individual. For example, pneumonia may not kill someone who has good health, but it can be deadly to someone who is HIV-positive. Additionally, someone who is HIV-positive may easily contract viruses and bacterial infections much more easily than someone with good health, even if they are not sexually active following their diagnosis.

Apple cider vinegar does not cure AIDS itself, nor does it cure anyone who is HIV-positive. What it does do, however, is ease the discomfort and pain associated with being HIV-positive. It has also helped people to tolerate their medications and the medicinal cocktails they must ingest as part of their treatment by alleviating digestional discomfort.

Studies have found that apple cider vinegar alone will not help people who are HIV-positive. Anyone who is HIV-positive who is interested in using apple cider vinegar for relief will need to combine the vinegar with other products. One of these products is bee propolis, which is sold in health food stores. Bee propolis is a non-toxic beehive product and it is safe for ingestion. It has been found to contain elements that are used in medications given to patients who are HIV-positive. These elements are known to inhibit the growth of HIV. Additionally, people have found that adding cayenne pepper to their treatment has also been helpful in combatting the negative side effects of being HIV-positive, as well as the sickness they often experience from the medications. For best results, take the cayenne pepper as a supplement. It is also a good idea to drink more water than normal during this treatment, preferably 4 liters of water a day.

While consuming apple cider vinegar will not "cure" someone of AIDS, it can be a potent fighter against the HIV virus. This is especially true if taken with bee propolis. All the same, just as it does with cancer, apple cider vinegar will boost the alkalinity of your body, an environment that the HIV virus cannot thrive in. As this occurs, the virus will weaken. Also, the HIV virus stays strong in the body by encasing itself in what is known as a "lipid envelope." This is how it wards off attacks from white blood cells, the body's natural defense against any infection. The acetic acid in apple cider vinegar has been found to attack lipids, thereby destroying these protective envelopes the virus tries to hide in. The more these protective casings are torn away thanks to apple cider vinegar, the more vulnerable the virus becomes to white blood cells. Thus, the virus is slowed down from spreading.

There have been many reports from people who are HIV-positive finding relief from some of the negative side effects of their condition thanks to apple cider vinegar.

One negative side effect of being HIV-positive is constant vomiting. In just such a case, the person found relief after consuming either white vinegar or apple cider vinegar. For a person who is unable to keep anything down (including their medication), it's worth giving apple cider vinegar a try. It will alleviate the digestive problems and make it easier for a person to be able to eat again without the worry of bringing everything back up again.

Other patients diagnosed as HIV-positive have also reported relief from other negative side effects after they added apple cider vinegar to their diet. One person suffering from constipation reported that all was right again after they started consuming apple cider vinegar. Another who experienced stomach upset and painful bowel movements eventually found relief after including apple cider vinegar in his diet. Apple cider vinegar has been found to ease these types of discomfort, as well as many others that are just as harsh to go through when someone is HIV-positive. Apple cider vinegar has been found to detox the colon and improve intestinal health, so this may be why it is such a good idea to use it for stomach and bowel problems.

There has definitely been a lot of progress in treating patients diagnosed as HIV-positive with apple cider vinegar. It will take time for it to work, but if a person is interested in using ACV to combat the negative effects of their disease, and can stick to a regimen, the results will be well worth the wait.

For best results, choose any one of these treatments. If you are not sure about using any one of these treatments, talk with your doctor first. Explore your options and decide if this would be a good choice for you in treating HIV. If anything, it is worth a try to alleviate the intestinal discomfort and allow you to be able to take your medication without worry.

When using any one of these suggested methods of including apple cider vinegar in your diet, be sure to combine the suggested doses with 2 capsules each of cayenne pepper and bee propolis.

1. Take two ACV supplements three times a day every 8 hours.

2. Consume one tablespoon of ACV three times a day.

3. Add 2 tablespoons of ACV to a glass of water and drink 3 times a day, preferably 8 hours apart.

4. Add apple cider vinegar to your diet by eating it on your salads, as a pickled egg or with other meals.

Apple cider vinegar has so many healing properties in it that it can certainly be useful in treating the negative side effects and symptoms of those who are HIV-positive. When other kinds of medications cannot help alleviate the digestional problems preventing these patients from taking their medications, apple cider vinegar becomes a good choice and just may help these patients find the relief they need.

Keep in mind that the positive results from including apple cider vinegar in your diet may not bring the same satisfaction to you as it has done for other people. Give it some time to work and decide if this is best for you. If you feel that apple cider vinegar would be a wise choice to add to your treatment of being HIV-positive, discuss this with your doctor and keep track of your progress. Ultimately, consuming apple cider vinegar can boost your health and it may hopefully help you in the fight against AIDS.

How to Use Apple Cider Vinegar for Weight Loss

If your goal is to lose weight, it might be a good idea to add apple cider vinegar to your diet. There's a lot of speculation floating around over whether or not it can help you lose weight, and a lot of so-called "experts" may be putting down apple cider vinegar for weight loss on one hand and then urging you to try their product on the other hand. A lot of people in the medical community may believe and even preach that apple cider vinegar is not helpful in the battle to lose weight, but a lot of evidence would point otherwise.

So have people actually lost weight when using apple cider vinegar? Indeed, they have. Reports of how people have lost weight after using apple cider vinegar are all over the Internet. Granted, you must take everything you read with a grain of salt, but those who have shared their stories of how apple cider vinegar has helped them lose weight are backing up their claims with further evidence of lifestyle changes. We'll get more into these changes soon.

It is no surprise that apple cider vinegar has helped people to lose weight. It is perhaps one of the most natural power-packed ingredients on the market which can help people in a variety of ways. Weight loss is just one of these ways. Apple cider vinegar actually works to help fight fat because of its natural effect on the body and digestive system. There are 3 ways in which apple cider vinegar can help you lose weight:

1. Apple cider vinegar naturally boosts metabolism

2. Apple cider vinegar attacks fat.

3. The acetic acid in apple cider vinegar may prevent the digestion of starch.

These actions make it a great tool to use for weight loss. On top of this, apple cider vinegar will eventually give you more energy, making you feel ready for exercise when you would have otherwise been too tired to even walk up a flight of stairs. Adding vinegar to your diet will also make you feel fuller sooner than with other meals. This is especially true if you eat a high-carb meal with the apple cider vinegar. By feeling full sooner, you'll end up eating less.

The key to using apple cider vinegar for weight loss is not just to rely on swallowing a couple of tablespoons a day and hoping the pounds will just magically melt off. It takes more than a "magic ingredient" to ensure you will lose weight. There have certainly been positive results when people used apple cider vinegar to help them shed the pounds, but they have also made other dietary changes, as well as lifestyle changes. If you want to try using apple cider vinegar to help you lose weight, you will need to make these changes, too.

One such change you will need to make if you want to use apple cider vinegar for weight loss is to be more active. If you are not exercising for at least a half hour every day, start doing so. The biggest struggle in fitting exercise into our lives is having the time. Life is too busy to exercise. But try squeezing in a workout or a walk early in the morning, during your lunch break or after dinner. Instead of watching TV or surfing the Internet, exercise instead. There are many books out there you can check out on how to fit an exercise routine into your busy life.

Another change you'll have to make when using apple cider vinegar for weight loss is to your diet and eating habits. You'll need to start opting for healthier, low-fat foods, as well as practicing portion control.

A third change you will need to make in using apple cider vinegar for weight loss is to include a food journal. Writing down everything you eat – including snacks – will make you more aware of what you are eating and how many calories you consume each day. By studying your food journal, you'll start becoming more aware of your food choices and when you'll need to start making healthier ones.

Finally, as with all methods used for weight loss, implementing apple cider vinegar in your diet as part of your effort to lose weight will require time and patience. It will not start working overnight. You will need to give it some time before you notice any results. Most people have found that it took a few months before they noticed the weight going down.

Ready to start using apple cider vinegar for weight loss? If so, you will not need to start buying tons of bottles of apple cider vinegar at the store or adding it to everything you eat. You can most certainly add apple cider vinegar, or any other vinegar, to foods such as salads and meat marinades, but the one way to use it for weight loss is very simple: Just stir two tablespoons of apple cider vinegar into an 8-ounce glass of water and drink it before meals. That's all there is to it. If you prefer, add a teaspoon of organic honey for better taste, or add the apple cider vinegar to a glass of orange juice. Following this routine will help you bring apple cider vinegar into your diet and soon you will start experiencing the other health benefits ACV can give to you in your fight against the extra weight.

When using apple cider vinegar for weight loss in conjunction with other changes, it's important to note that you will need to keep the ACV in the program. Studies of people who successfully used apple cider vinegar for weight loss found that the people gained all the weight back once they stopped consuming the vinegar and went back to their dormant habits. If you want to keep using apple cider vinegar as part of a weight loss plan, you will need to make it a part of your routine in the long term. That said, apple cider vinegar has many other health benefits, so you can at least look forward to enjoying a healthier life after becoming a "new you." If you wish, you can decrease the amount of apple cider vinegar you consume with each meal to one teaspoon instead of two tablespoons.

While using apple cider vinegar for weight loss, make sure you check in with your doctor, nutritionist or dietitian every once in a while. Keep an eye on your progress and watch out for any negative side effects or health conditions flaring up. Apple cider vinegar can indeed help you lose weight when used correctly, and keeping it as part of your weight loss routine will create long-term benefits for you both in losing weight and in your quest to live a healthier life.

Beauty Uses for Apple Cider Vinegar

Apple cider vinegar has helped many people experience a variety of benefits on the inside, but guess what? It can also help you experience benefits on the outside, too. From the inside and out, apple cider vinegar has a way of making a person "right again" and, ultimately, beautiful. There are quite a few beauty benefits you can achieve just from using apple cider vinegar. Additionally, many people have found that it works much better than products sold on store shelves.

You can rest easy using apple cider vinegar for your beauty routine, knowing that you are using an all-natural product straight from the planet. What's more, you won't go broke using apple cider vinegar as part of your beauty routine, because since you only need a little of it at a time, that large bottle of ACV can last you a lot longer.

Here is a list of the many ways apple cider vinegar can promote hair and skin health. It can also create more beautiful teeth and feet. Once you start using apple cider vinegar for your beauty routine, keep in mind that it will take time before you notice results. You can alternate using apple cider vinegar with other products or using it once a week. In some cases, you may need to use it every day. Read the instructions carefully and see if this method works for you.

Fights dandruff

Apple cider vinegar gets a lot of grief for being acidic, but for once, being acidic is beneficial when dealing with dandruff. The acidic level balances the pH level of your scalp, helping to ward of any fungal growth and strengthening your scalp's protective mantel layer. There are two ways you can use apple cider vinegar to fight dandruff. One way is to mix equal parts of apple cider vinegar with water and massaging it into your hair before your shower. Make sure it has contact with your scalp and you really massage it onto there. Allow it to set for a few minutes then rinse. Shampoo and condition your hair as normal. The other way to use apple cider vinegar to treat dandruff is to add a teaspoon of apple cider vinegar to your shampoo then using as normal, making sure you rub it onto your scalp. Rinse then use conditioner as directed.

Tones skin

A whole host of environmental factors can damage your skin. From dust to pollutants to even the air you breathe, your skin is constantly under attack. During this process, the strength and pH level of your skin can weaken, making it flabby and unattractive. To restore this pH balance and make your skin stronger, if not shinier, try using apple cider vinegar. Here again, there are two ways to use it to tone your skin. First, add one cup of apple cider vinegar to your bath water and soak in the tub for 15 minutes. Second, mix one part of apple cider vinegar with 2 parts of water and use a cotton ball dipped into this solution to dab on the "T-zone" of your face (the forehead, nose and your chin).

Fights acne

Using apple cider vinegar for facial treatment will strengthen your skin, kill dead skin cells and promote a healthier pH level of your skin. But if you see a breakout, treat it right away with apple cider vingar. Here again, there are two methods that have been proven to work. One way to use apple cider vinegar to treat acne is to simply soak a cottonball in apple cider vinegar then dab it onto the affected area before bedtime. Rinse the area in the morning and the acne should be gone. Another way to use apple cider vinegar for this purpose is to combine 1 part of vinegar to 4 quarts of water and use a cottonball dipped in this solution to apply to the area. Leave it on for 10 minutes then rinse. You will need to repeat this method three times a day to see results.

Promotes foot beauty and health

Apple cider vinegar has helped people improve their foot health and create more attractive feet. In addition to being used to treat athlete's foot, it has been found to create softer, cleaner and smoother skin on the feet. It can also get rid of toe fungus. Another bonus is that it can eliminate nasty foot odors. To get this benefit simply soak your feet in a solution of 1 cup of apple cider vinegar added to 4 cups of water for at least 15 minutes. Then rinse your feet and dry.

Reduces varicose veins

Apple cider vinegar improves circulation and blood flow in the veins, making it an ideal candidate for fighting varicose veins. Varicose veins occur when the valves in your veins weaken, causing them to become enlarged or tangled. This can stop blood flow through that area, causing painful cramping or blood clots. They usually happen in the legs and they are most prominent during old age. Since apple cider vinegar can help reduce this kind of problem, it can be useful in fighting varicose veins and keeping your blood flow going strong. To use for this purpose, add one part of apple cider vinegar to one part of a body lotion and rub over the area twice a day.

Gets rid of age spots

There's no question that apple cider vinegar is good for your skin. Time and again, it has been proven to help create healthier, shinier skin. Part of this treatment includes tackling skin problems such as scaly patches, liver spots and age spots. To use, soak a cottonball in apple cider vinegar then dab the area before bedtime. Rinse the area in the morning. If using pure apple cider vinegar on the skin stings, dilute the ACV with water. If you want to get rid of these unattractive skin blemishes on the hands or feet, you can soak them in a bowl of apple cider vinegar for at least 15 minutes then rinsing and drying. Also, you can add water to these soaks if it irritates the skin.

Promotes soft and shiny hair

The acetic acid in apple cider vinegar has helped many people find it to be a great benefit for hair health. It has helped promote hair growth, fight dandruff, clean your scalp of any build-up left over from hair care products and create stronger hair. In fact, it has also helped get rid of split ends. There are two ways you can use apple cider vinegar for your hair health. One method is to apply ½ cup to 1 cup of apple cider vinegar (depending on your hair length) to your hair, massaging it into your scalp, then wrapping it in a shower cap or towel and leaving it on for 10 minutes before showering. Rinse hair thoroughly before shampooing. Another method is to add 1/3 cup of the vinegar to 4 cups of water then pouring it over your hair after you shampoo it. Leave it in your hair for a few seconds before rinsing with cold water. Apply conditioner as directed.

Promotes hair growth

Apple cider vinegar will stimulate the growth of hair follicles. It will also ease an itchy, dry scalp. To use for hair growth, add 1 part apple cider vinegar to 1 part warm water. Apply to your hair after you shampoo and leave it in a couple of minutes. Rinse from hair completely then continue your hair-washing routine. For best results, use this method once a week.

Facial mask

As mentioned, apple cider vinegar is great for cleaner, healthier skin. One way you can use apple cider vinegar for skin health is to create a facial mask. To do this, you will need to mix equal parts of apple cider vinegar with bentonite clay and add 1 tablespoon of raw honey. Apply this to your face and leave it on for 10-15 minutes. Rinse with warm water and pat skin dry. Use once a day, preferably in the morning.

Facial scrub

Want to use apple cider vinegar as a facial wash? Since it's good for your skin, there's no harm in giving it a try. To use for a facial scrub, add 1 tablespoon of apple cider vinegar to 2 cups of warm water. Dab the area with a cotton ball or splash onto your face.

Whitens teeth

Even though apple cider vinegar is acidic, many people have found that it can help them whiten their teeth. To get this benefit, gargle with apple cider vinegar before brushing your teeth. Because it can damage tooth enamel, use only a little bit of the vinegar.

Fights cellulite

Nothing says "yucky" like flabby cellulite on the legs and arms. You can combat this unattractive skin condition with apple cider vinegar. Add 1 cup of apple cider vinegar to a warm bath and soak for a half hour.

Apple cider vinegar can certainly be added to your beauty routine. You may need to alternate its use or change how much of it you use, but once implemented, it can help you achieve more attractive and healthier results for your skin and hair.

How to Detox with Apple Cider Vinegar

People have been using apple cider vinegar for a variety of reasons for years. As an antiseptic, cleaning solution, beauty aid and health remedy, apple cider vinegar has proven to be a natural remedy for a variety of ailments. It also works well as a detox aid.

Now more than ever, our bodies are exposed to a variety of toxins. From the food we eat to the air we breathe, harmful toxins get into our bodies and wreak havoc on our health. To get rid of the toxins, we can use a process known as "detoxification," or "detox" for short. By going through the process of detoxing our bodies, we remove those harmful substances and give our bodies a stronger fighting chance in combatting disease and sickness. What's more, detoxing the body has given many people a new burst of energy and a sense of starting anew.

What better choice than to use apple cider vinegar for a detox purpose? It has a variety of benefits and can help you get rid of negative toxins. As to how often you should use apple cider vinegar for detox purposes, you can do so once a month, one whole month, or daily. This is a personal choice and it must be based on your own convenience, taste preference and lifestyle.

How exactly can apple cider vinegar help you to detox? For one thing, it kills harmful bacteria in your body. It also destroys fungus and prevents the spread of certain diseases. It breaks down mucus build-up and purifies your blood. Here are the things that can happen when you use apple cider vinegar for detox purposes:

- Cleans out the colon

- Cleanses the liver

- Cleanses the kidneys

- Clears the lymph nodes

- Clears the intestines.

What's more, apple cider vinegar is packed with powerful vitamins and enzymes. You'll be doing your body a favor in using apple cider vinegar for detox purposes because you'll also be giving it a good boost in overall health.

There are two ways you can detox with apple cider vinegar. One way is to drink it and another way is to use it in a bath. For best results, use both methods, as the detox bath is mostly for detoxing your skin and not so much for the inside of your body.

There are a variety of "apple cider vinegar detox drinks" that can be found on the Internet. In fact, you may even find it already put together as a mix or as a tea bag sold in the store. Take some time going over the many recipes available and see which one you would like to try. If one drink doesn't work out for you, try another one. There are a few included in this book but you can find many others on the Internet. You may also come across an apple cider vinegar cookbook that may contain a recipe for a detox drink.

Before you use apple cider vinegar as a drink, remember that you should never drink apple cider vinegar without adding it to another liquid first, such as water or juice.

If you would like to detox with apple cider vinegar in a drink, you can drink it cold or as a hot tea. For the cold drink, mix together a tablespoon of apple cider vinegar, the juice from a lemon, 1/8 teaspoon of cayenne pepper or cinnamon and 2 tablespoons of raw honey in ¼ cup of water. Drink daily, preferably in the morning before breakfast. You can also add 2 tablespoons of apple cider vinegar to a water bottle containing 2 liters of filtered water and sip this all day long. As a hot tea, add 2 tablespoons of apple cider vinegar to a 16-ounce mug of warm water. Add 2 tablespoons of raw honey, lemon juice and a pinch of cayenne pepper or cinnamon.

You can also use an apple cider detox bath to help remove toxins from your skin. To detox in the bath, fill your bathtub with very warm water. Add 4 ounces of apple cider vinegar, 2 cups of baking soda and 2 cups of Epsom salt. Swirl the water in a circle so that it is all mixed together really well. Soak in the water for at least a half hour then pat yourself dry.

Apple cider vinegar has a variety of natural bacteria fighters that can help you remove harmful toxins from your body. Once you go through the detox episode, you'll feel a lot "lighter" and healthier. For best results, try to include as much organic and raw, wholesome foods in your diet to keep that detox effect and avoid ingesting more harmful toxins.

Try using apple cider vinegar for your next detox episode and watch just how healthier and happier you'll start to feel.

The Side Effects of Using Apple Cider Vinegar

As with everything on the market out there, even things that are natural and straight from the earth, there can be negative side effects associated with using apple cider vinegar. This book has provided you with clear instructions on the many ways to use apple cider vinegar, as well as reminders on how not to use it. All the same, we will go over what can go wrong if apple cider vinegar is not used correctly. While the focus will be on internal use, we'll also touch on how it can cause negative effects when used topically or as a cleaning solution.

Some people have used apple cider vinegar for helping their pets when the animals are experiencing health problems. While apple cider vinegar is safe for pet ingestion, it is really a good idea to practice caution before administering it to your animal friend. Just as apple cider vinegar is not for everyone, it's not for every animal, either. What may work for one animal, even one of the same species, may not work for another. There is the risk that you may give your animal friend too much apple cider vinegar, or you may give it to them the wrong way. After ingesting apple cider vinegar, your pet may experience negative side effects ranging from diarrhea, constipation, sensitive teeth and kidney problems. It can also cause the animal to experience sensitivity of the mouth. One other factor to be aware of before giving your pet apple cider vinegar is that there is a possibility your pet is allergic to apple cider vinegar. If this is the case and you give your pet the apple cider vinegar, he or she may vomit it right back up. Your best bet is to consult with a veterinarian before giving apple cider vinegar to your pet to determine if there is an allergy to it.

If you are already taking medication, use caution before you start drinking or taking apple cider vinegar. Studies have shown that apple cider vinegar works against certain medications. Thus far reported, it's not advisable to consume apple cider vinegar if you are on medication for heart disease or diabetes. Also, the apple cider vinegar will counteract the effects of laxatives or diuretics. It can also lower the potassium levels in your body, so if you are already taking medication specifically for this purpose, avoid consuming apple cider vinegar until you finish using the medication. If you're not sure if it's safe to consume apple cider vinegar while on medication, discuss this with your doctor first.

Pregnant or nursing woman may also want to use caution before adding apple cider vinegar to their diets. There have not been enough studies performed to determine if apple cider vinegar is safe during pregnancy. Also, if ingesting the vinegar or taking the supplements, it can pass through the breast milk. Again, discuss this with your doctor before adding apple cider vinegar to your diet.

Drinking the apple cider vinegar without diluting it first has been found to create a variety of negative side effects. It's really not a good idea to drink it raw. Always dilute it in a liquid first. If you drink raw apple cider without diluting it, and especially if you do this often enough, these are the types of negative side effects that can happen:

- Sore throat

- Tooth decay or damage

- Upset stomach

- Nausea

- Tooth decay

To avoid these effects, always dilute the ACV before drinking it. And to protect your teeth, always drink ACV drinks with a straw.

Raw apple cider can also cause problems when applied to the skin. Here again, always dilute it first or add other ingredients, such as baking soda. Some people who applied undiluted apple cider vinegar to their skin with a cloth or poultice or left it on for an hour or more experienced rashes or burning of the skin. Never wash your skin with raw apple cider or treat any part of your body with a raw apple cider wash. If you must use it, do so only for a few seconds then rinse with water.

While apple cider vinegar has a variety of health and beauty benefits, it is not for everyone. In fact, some people may actually be allergic to apple cider vinegar. If you are unsure about whether or not you are allergic to apple cider vinegar, or any vinegar, start with a very small amount, such as a teaspoon in a glass of water or as a topical solution included in this book. Common symptoms of an allergic reaction to apple cider vinegar include a rash, shortness of breath, and itching. If you experience any of these symptoms after only using a small amount of apple cider vinegar either orally or topically, stop use immediately.

Some people use apple cider vinegar for detox purposes. During the detox period, you may experience a headache as your body is working to get rid of the harmful toxins. This is a natural reaction. However, if the headache is too severe or if it doesn't go away after a few days, stop the detox method immediately and you should find relief soon.

While the lowering of blood sugar levels can be a good thing for most folks who are trying to avoid being diagnosed with Type 2 Diabetes, this is not such good news for anyone who is already diagnosed or who has insulin resistance. By constantly lowering blood sugar levels, apple cider vinegar can cause the body to go into a state of diabetic hypoglycemia, thereby depriving the brain of glucose. A person who has reached this point may begin to experience seizures or lose consciousness. If you have been diagnosed with diabetes, it is strongly recommended that you consult with your doctor before adding apple cider vinegar to your regimen. A little apple cider vinegar on your salad or in your food is fine, but too much, and especially long-term, can be deadly. Follow your doctor's medication and treatment instructions before making any changes.

Another way in which apple cider vinegar has been used for health benefits is as an enema. In this case, there can be negative side effects as well. A lot of cider vinegar proponents have shared how this use has been great and wonderful for them, but other people are not so adept at creating their own enemas or using them have experienced negative, even painful, effects. When used incorrectly, they have experienced a damaged spincter or blood in the stool following the procedure. It is a good idea to seek out a homeopathic practitioner or an herbalist instead of creating a DIY apple cider vinegar enema. It is also recommended that a licensed physician should administer the enema.

On a final note, watch out for imitations of apple cider vinegar or those sold without the "Mother" included. These are not very effective brands of apple cider vinegar and usually will not give you the same health benefits as the kind that is raw, organic and contains the "Mother." You can find this kind of apple cider vinegar at most grocery stores as well as larger stores in your area. Make sure you buy and use the same good quality apple cider vinegar that most people have come to know and trust. The imitation brands may be more affordable or available, but they will not work as effectively.

While you are using apple cider vinegar, keep a close eye on the positive and negative effects you experience from it. If possible, keep a journal. Let your doctor know you have added it to your diet and stop use immediately if severe or emergency symptoms arise. For the most part, apple cider vinegar is safe for consumption, but keep in mind the proper way of using it so you can avoid any negative side effects or problems.

www.ingramcontent.com/pod-product-compliance
Lightning Source LLC
Chambersburg PA
CBHW062018280526
45787CB00005B/2152